Secret to Women's Longevity?

By

Lucy Becker

Table of Contents

Introduction

Have you ever wondered why males typically live shorter lives than women? What keeps them going for so long? We'll look at the many aspects, such as heredity, dietary practices, and environmental variables, that affect how long women live. We'll also talk about the difficulties elderly women have keeping up their health and well-being and offer solutions. On average, women live longer than men do throughout the world, and scientists have generally linked these sex-based differences in lifespan to biological variables that affect survival. *A recent study of wild mammals revealed significant differences in longevity and aging in several mammalian species.* Women typically live around 10% longer than men do in humans. But among wild mammals, several of the species examined females typically have varied mammal groupings and have very varied ratios. You should read this book if you want to find out more about the scientific basis for women living longer lives and if you also want to increase your health and longevity as a woman. *Academics, researchers, and health enthusiasts have been baffled by this question for many years.* It has been the subject of numerous research to try and explain why women often live longer than males. In this book, we'll look into the science of women's health and welfare as well as the elements that affect women's longevity. *Hendrikje Van Andel-Schipper gave longevity researchers a perfect example of how women live longer lives than men when their body is tested by scientists.* When she passed away at the age of 115, she was the oldest person in the world, and a team of Dutch researchers used her body to conduct some ground-breaking studies on why some women live longer than others. In 2010, researchers at the VU University Medical Center in Amsterdam, under the direction of Dr. Henne Holstege, sequenced Andel-Schipper's DNA to learn more about the mechanisms underlying long life. In the most recent investigation, *the scientists examined Andel-Schipper's blood for gene alterations.* White blood cells, for example, are produced by stem cells during division. They sought to ascertain whether healthy white blood cells can develop mutations over time and whether these changes have any effects on health. Even though she was generally healthy, they found hundreds of genetic changes in her cells, which they found to be odd. So the scientists looked at her stem cells and tried to figure out where these white blood cells were originating from. Every person is thought to have roughly *20,000 stem cells at birth, of which about 1,300 are active. Andel-Schipper had only two active stem cells at the time of her death, which surprised the researchers.* When the telomeres on Andel-Schipper's blood cells were measured, the researchers found that they were incredibly short when compared to all of her other organs. Telomeres shorten as cells get older. As a result, the scientists concluded that women's stem cells may have a maximum number of divisions they can make before beginning to die as a result of division exhaustion.

The researchers acknowledge that more research is required to ascertain whether stem cell exhaustion was the cause of Andel-Schipper's death and whether it could also be the cause of death in women who live to a ripe old age. If confirmed, there are important consequences for aging. Therefore, even though there are probably multiple overlapping factors at work, a recent study reveals that stem cells may be one of the keys to a longer life for women. The three main factors that affect lifespan are genetics, environment, and lifestyle. But we do have some degree of control over our way of life. According to research, thinking and acting with optimism will help you generally expect good things to happen in the future. Actionable science The Women's Health Initiative is a long-term study that started in 1993 and is still operating today. The researchers used data from this study. They specifically collected data from over 159,255 study participants, who ranged in age from 50 to over 80. After enrolling more women in 2000 they monitored each one for up to several years. The results of the participant's responses were then used to establish a score. *Demographics, chronic illness, depression, and other health-related characteristics were all controlled for by the researchers.* The relationship between optimism and lifespan persisted even after considering these variables. Women live longer than males around the world, but this wasn't always the case. According to the data from wealthy nations. Why do women currently live longer than males, and why has this benefit grown over time? We just have fragmentary evidence and responses. We are aware that the longer life expectancy of women than that of men is influenced by *biological, behavioral, and environmental factors.* Regardless of the precise weight, we know that several significant non-biological elements have changed, which may account for at least some of the reasons why women live so much longer than males do today but did not in the past. What are these altering variables? Some of these are well-known and rather simple, like the fact that men smoke more frequently. Some are trickier than others. There is evidence, for instance, that in wealthy nations the female advantage increased in part because, in the past, *infectious diseases disproportionately affected women. As a result, medical advancements that lessened the long-term health burden of infectious diseases especially for survivors ended up raising women's longevity disproportionately.* According to the data, there are chromosomal and hormonal differences between men and women that have an impact on longevity. For instance, men often have more visceral fat (**fat that surrounds the organs**) but women typically have more subcutaneous fat (**fat that sits directly under the skin**). This variation, which affects longevity since fat around the organs is a predictor of *cardiovascular disease in females*, is influenced by both estrogen and the existence of the second X chromosome.

However, biological variations can only be a part of the tale; otherwise, we wouldn't notice such significant variations through time and across nations. What else might be happening, we do have some hints. For instance, we are aware that changes in men's smoking patterns have impacted mortality trends. Additionally, we are aware that historical medical advancements have had varied effects on men's and women's health outcomes.

Chapter 1

The Biology of Women's Longevity

Women frequently outlive men, and the causes are complex and multifaceted. Due to some biological and environmental factors, women often live longer than men. Cardiovascular disease is one of the major causes, and women are less prone than males to develop it. This might be a result of estrogen's protective qualities, which have been shown to improve blood vessel health, boost cholesterol levels, and reduce inflammation. Another factor is that women have stronger immune systems than men, giving them a higher chance of fighting off infections. This may be because estrogen activates the immune system and is found in larger concentrations in women. women are less prone to develop particular diseases like lung and colon cancer. Changes in lifestyle and behavior, as well as hormonal factors, maybe to fault. Women may be more adept at managing stress than men. Variations in coping strategies, as well as brain structure and function, may be to blame for this. a distinction that appears to apply to females and males in the animal kingdom. Why is this the situation? *Genetically, the majority of men have an X and a Y chromosome, while the majority of women have two X chromosomes. X chromosomes are home to thousands of genes that produce proteins*, but Y chromosomes, despite having less *genetic material, contain the gene that controls masculine* characteristics like the growth of the testes. This gene is known as "**SRY**."Women often live longer than men, according to existing studies, and this pattern is seen in many mammals, where females outlast males.No one is yet certain why this is the case, but a recent study conducted by scientists at the *University of California, San Francisco (UCSF)* may now provide a reason. Discovery Series of the XX chromosomal pairing has genetic material that can lengthen longevity, but only in the presence of corresponding female hormones, which the ovaries secrete, according to Trusted Source, which is featured in the journal Aging Cell and is available to read online.

*Genetics and the length of life in women

There is ongoing research into how genetics affect women's longevity. The age at which women may encounter age-related diseases and death appears to be greatly influenced by genetics, even while lifestyle factors like food and exercise are known to play a considerable effect on overall health and lifespan.

According to studies, some genetic variants may be linked to longer lifespans in women. For instance, certain mutations in the **FOXO3 gene**, which is involved in cellular maintenance and repair, have been linked to a longer life expectancy in women. Additional research has also shown certain genetic variations that may be linked to a lower risk of age-related illnesses like cancer and cardiovascular disease. For instance, changes in the **BRCA1** and **BRCA2** genes have been associated with a reduced risk of breast and ovarian cancer, two diseases that can significantly increase a woman's mortality. It's crucial to remember that lifestyle factors like diet, exercise, refraining from smoking, and excessive alcohol consumption can have a big impact on general health and longevity. Genetics is only one component in lifespan determination. In addition, long life is not guaranteed by heredity, and some environmental factors can significantly affect health and lifespan.

***The effects of hormones on the health of women**

Women's health is greatly influenced by hormones, which have an impact on both their *physical and emotional well-being. The menstrual cycle is regulated by hormones, especially estrogen, and progesterone.* These hormones play a role in regulating ovulation, the formation of the uterine lining, and the frequency and length of menstruation. *Hormonal abnormalities can result in irregular menstrual cycles, excessive bleeding, and excruciating cramps.* For female reproduction, hormones are essential. *The luteinizing hormone (LH) and follicle-stimulating hormone (FSH) stimulate the release of eggs from the ovaries and control the menstrual cycle. For a healthy pregnancy to continue, estrogen and progesterone are necessary.* To maintain women's bone density, estrogen is essential. Estrogen levels decrease as women become older and enter menopause, which can cause osteoporosis and bone loss. A woman's emotions and mood might be affected by hormonal changes. *For instance, premenstrual syndrome (PMS) symptoms such as mood swings, irritability,* and anxiety can be brought on by low estrogen and progesterone levels during the menstrual cycle. Depression and anxiety can both be exacerbated by hormonal abnormalities. *The metabolism is greatly influenced by hormones including insulin, thyroid hormone, and cortisol.* Metabolic diseases, insulin resistance, and weight gain can all be caused by hormonal imbalances. Hormones can impact various aspects of skin health, such as acne, hair growth, and skin aging.

As an illustration, unwanted hair growth and acne can both be brought on by high levels of androgens (**male hormones**). The health of women is greatly influenced by hormones, which affect everything from reproductive function to mood, metabolism, and skin health. It's crucial to maintain hormonal balance through healthy lifestyle choices and, when necessary, medical treatment because hormonal imbalances can cause a variety of health issues.

Chapter 2

Lifestyle and Longevity

*Sleep patterns and the effect on female longevity

Women's longevity may be significantly impacted by their sleep patterns. According to research, having adequate good sleep is crucial for preserving health and lowering one's chance of developing some conditions, *including heart disease, stroke, diabetes, and obesity*. Lack of sleep has been associated with a reduced life expectancy and a higher risk of developing chronic illnesses like cancer. Compared to women who get seven to eight hours of sleep per night, those who routinely obtain less than six hours of sleep each night are more likely to experience these health issues. Longevity also depends on the quality of sleep. Chronic health issues may be more likely to affect women who frequently encounter sleep disturbances or who have a sleep disorder like sleep apnea. Age, hormonal changes during menopause, and lifestyle elements like stress, exercise, and diet can also affect how much and how well women sleep. Women who put a high priority on healthy sleep practices including creating a regular sleep schedule, a soothing nighttime routine, and avoiding gadgets before bed are more likely to live longer, healthier lives. In general, if you want to maximize your health and lifespan as a woman, you must prioritize developing appropriate sleep habits. Women can decrease their chance of developing chronic health issues and live longer, healthier lives by prioritizing sleep and taking action to enhance its quality and length.

*Women's social networks and mental health

Women's mental health can be significantly impacted by their social networks. *According to research, women who are socially connected and have a support network typically experience better mental health results than their socially isolated counterparts.* One explanation for this is the sense of belonging that comes from social ties, which has been shown to improve emotions of contentment and well-being. Women who feel socially connected are also more likely to be able to get emotional assistance, which can aid them in managing stress and challenging circumstances. *Additionally, social contacts can give women the chance to follow their interests and hobbies,* which can enhance their general quality of life and raise their self-esteem. Women who don't have many social relationships, on the other hand, may feel depressed, lonely, and alone.

Numerous detrimental health effects, including an elevated risk for mental health conditions like anxiety and depression, may result from this. It is evident that when it comes to women's mental health, social ties are a crucial component to take into account. Women can have happier, healthier lives by developing and maintaining strong social networks.

Chapter 3

Cultural Aspects and the Longevity of Women

*The influence of tradition and culture on women's health

Women's health outcomes can be significantly influenced by culture and customs. Women's perceptions of and approaches to managing their health, access to healthcare services, and interactions with healthcare professionals can all be influenced by cultural and traditional ideas, practices, and values. Women's health is directly related to their role in reproduction in many cultures, and hence, concerns about reproductive health may be stigmatized or taboo. Women may feel too humiliated or embarrassed to seek medical attention for problems relating to their reproductive health, such as *menstruation, contraception, or STDs*, as a result of this. Women may experience pressure in some societies to put the needs of their families before their own, which can result in neglecting their health. Women's health results might also be affected by conventional medical procedures like herbal medicines or spiritual therapy. While some traditional practices may be helpful, others might be dangerous or ineffectual, especially if they are employed in place of medical therapies that are supported by evidence. Women's health can also be impacted by cultural and conventional gender roles and expectations. Women are frequently expected to take on caregiving responsibilities in many cultures, which can lead to added stress, weariness, and a lack of time to attend to their own health needs. While making sure that women have access to accurate and thorough health information and healthcare services, *it is critical to understand and respect cultural and traditional beliefs and practices.* Healthcare professionals should aim to provide care that is sensitive to cultural differences and promote wellness by collaborating with women and their communities.

*The effects of gender roles on women's lives

The expectations that society and culture impose on people depending on their gender are known as gender roles. As they frequently specify what women are supposed to do and how they should behave in various spheres of their lives, these roles have a considerable impact on women's lives. The strain to live up to society's ideals of femininity is one of the most significant effects of gender roles on women's life. It can be difficult for women to express themselves and pursue their goals because they are frequently expected to be loving, emotional, and subservient. As a result, there may be fewer prospects for employment and higher education, as well as a decrease in confidence and self-esteem. The roles of women in the home are impacted by gender roles as well. The traditional role of women as primary caregivers and homemakers can restrict their capacity to pursue their passions and occupations. *This may lead to an unfair division of household duties and responsibilities,* which would place an unfair burden on women. Gender roles also contribute to violence and discrimination against women based on gender. The notion that men should be in positions of dominance while women should be subservient can result in the view that women are inferior, which can encourage sexual harassment, assault, and other acts of violence against women. Gender stereotypes have a big impact on women's life, limiting their chances and fostering inequity. To develop a more fair and just society for all genders, it is crucial to confront and alter existing positions.

***Historical elements that increased women's longevity**

The longevity of women has been influenced historically by a number of things. High maternal mortality rates have historically had a negative impact on the life expectancy of women. *However, improvements in medical technology,* access to healthcare, and prenatal care have drastically lowered maternal mortality rates in many regions of the world, which has led to longer life expectancies for women. Due to cultural and societal conventions that prioritized men's health and well-being over women's, women were more likely than men to experience malnutrition. Women had limited access to healthcare due to a number of factors, including *poverty, discrimination, a lack of education, and lack of access to food and other resources.* However, improvements in agriculture, food distribution, and nutrition education have led to better overall nutrition for women, leading to improved health outcomes and longer lifespans. The longevity and health of women have been markedly enhanced by increased access to *healthcare, particularly preventative care including vaccinations, screenings, and early treatments.* Women now have better access to education, work, and other opportunities as a result of the changing roles that they play in society, which has led to an increase in their life expectancy. Women were frequently exposed to hazardous working conditions in factories, mines, and other industries, which caused higher rates of occupational illnesses and injuries. Women are now more likely to have higher-paying jobs, access to resources, and greater autonomy. However, more attention to workplace safety and modifications to labor laws have made it possible to lessen these risks and enhance the health of women.

Chapter 4

Women's Health Impact

*Global Trends in Women's Health and Longevity

Women tend to live longer than men around the world, and several factors, including access to healthcare, education, economic possibilities, cultural customs, and lifestyle choices, can affect a woman's health and longevity. The average life expectancy for men and women worldwide *is 70.8 years and 75.6 years*, respectively, according to the **World Health Organization (WHO)**. The life expectancy of women varies significantly between various nations and areas, nevertheless. For instance, with an average life expectancy of 87 years, Japan leads the pack among developed nations, followed by *Spain, Switzerland, Singapore, and Italy. Contrarily, sub-Saharan African nations like Sierra Leone, Chad, and Central African Republic* have the lowest life expectancy for women, with the majority of them dying before reaching their mid-fifties. Women's health and longevity are significantly influenced by access to healthcare. In nations with robust healthcare systems, women have better access to prenatal care, maternity healthcare, and preventative healthcare services, which can result in reduced rates of maternal mortality and better overall health outcomes. Women's health and longevity are also influenced by economic opportunity and education. Access to education and work is associated with improved health outcomes and longer life expectancies for women. In addition, they are more likely to have access to tools that might help them make informed decisions about their health. The health and longevity of women can also be impacted by cultural customs and lifestyle decisions. For instance, women are often expected to put their family's needs ahead of their own in some cultures, which can result in a disregard for their health. The health and longevity of women can also be negatively impacted by lifestyle decisions including smoking, drinking, and eating poorly. Women's health and longevity can be increased globally by expanding women's access to economic, educational, and healthcare opportunities as well as by encouraging healthy lifestyle choices.

*Social and economic variables' effects on women's health and longevity

Women's health and longevity are significantly impacted by socioeconomics.

Socioeconomically disadvantaged women confront many difficulties that may harm their health and life expectancy. Access to healthcare is a significant aspect. Regular preventive treatment, such as cancer screenings and vaccines, may be less likely to be received by women with lower earnings or less access to health insurance. *This might cause missing or delayed diagnosis, which can result in more advanced disease and worse consequences.* The kinds of jobs and working circumstances that women have access to can also be influenced by socioeconomic variables, which may have an impact on their physical health. The likelihood of occupational dangers, such as exposure to chemicals, as well as physically demanding tasks, which can raise the risk of injury and chronic pain, is higher for women in lower-paying jobs. *Access to wholesome food, a secure place to live, and exposure to environmental toxins are additional factors that may have an impact on women's health and longevity.* Socioeconomic status might also have an impact on these variables; women with lower incomes are more likely to reside in areas with unfavorable environmental conditions and restricted access to nutritious meals. In general, eliminating socioeconomic inequality is a crucial step toward enhancing the health and longevity of women. *This covers laws and initiatives that deal with the availability of healthcare, education, and employment possibilities.* We can contribute to the development of a more equitable society that promotes the health and well-being of all women by striving to enhance the social determinants of health.

*Disparities in Women's Health

Women's health and quality of life are significantly impacted by health inequalities among women around the world. Socioeconomic class, education, culture, access to healthcare, and governmental policy are just a few of the variables that can explain these discrepancies. In low-income nations, women frequently bear a disproportionately heavy burden of infectious diseases like malaria, *TB, and HIV/AIDS.* Due to the lack of access to trained birth attendants and reproductive health services, maternal death rates are also much higher in these areas. Poor health outcomes for women in low-income nations are also influenced by undernourishment and a lack of access to clean water and sanitary facilities. *Non-communicable diseases like diabetes, cancer,* and heart disease are more common in women in middle-income nations, frequently as a result of bad eating habits, smoking, and lack of physical activity. For some groups of women, such as those who reside in rural areas or come from *underprivileged communities*, access to healthcare may also be restricted. While women generally have more socioeconomic positions, higher levels of education, and better access to healthcare in high-income countries, gaps remain. Women who come from underserved groups, such as indigenous peoples, may encounter difficulties getting medical care and have higher incidences of chronic illnesses including diabetes and heart disease. *In high-income nations, women are more likely to have mental health problems including sadness and anxiety.* A multifaceted strategy is needed to reduce health disparities among women, including expanding access to *healthcare, enhancing socioeconomic status and education, and removing societal and cultural barriers to care.*

Chapter 5

Future Prospects for Longevity in Women

*Potential Lifetime of Women

Future life expectancy increases for women are highly likely thanks to medical progress. *We may be able to better comprehend and treat diseases that disproportionately impact women, such as breast cancer, ovarian cancer, and osteoporosis, with continuous study and development in fields like personalized medicine, gene therapy, and regenerative medicine.*

Furthermore, advancements in technologies like telemedicine and wearable health monitoring devices may make it possible to detect diseases earlier and implement more preventative healthcare practices. Additionally, studies have indicated that some *lifestyle factors*, including adhering to a balanced diet and exercise routine, lowering stress levels, and forgoing dangerous habits like smoking and binge drinking, can also promote lifespan. Women may be better equipped to take care of their health and possibly live longer if they are more aware of and educated about these variables. Even though many people's quality of life and length of life can be improved by medical developments, it is vital to keep in mind that there may also be societal and ethical issues to take into account. *The distribution of these breakthroughs, for instance, may be affected by problems with healthcare access and affordability. There may also be discussions on the moral implications of extending human life as well as its potential effects on population increase and resource distribution.*

*The moral ramifications of lengthening human life

Various ethical questions are brought up by the idea of extending human lifespans. There are worries about the effects on society and the individual, even if many people would welcome the potential to live longer, healthier lives. There is a chance that if life extension technologies are created, they will only be accessible to the wealthy, escalating already existing inequities. *Governments and legislators must make sure that everyone, regardless of socioeconomic standing, has access to life-extension technologies.* Increased population due to longer life expectancies would certainly worsen problems like climate change, resource depletion, and food shortages.

While it may be desired to live longer, it is also important to consider how well those extra years will be spent. Technologies for extending life should be created with an emphasis on raising the standard of living in old age rather than just extending it. Our perspectives on life, work, and relationships may alter as a result of life extension. For instance, people might decide to put off retiring, which would make the employment market more competitive. Furthermore, when people live longer and outlast their partners or children, relationships may become more complicated. Philosophical issues regarding the purpose of existence, the worth of time, and the certainty of death are brought up by the possibility of immortality. Some contend that being immortal could sap one's motivation, while others are concerned about the psychological effects of living forever. The subject of increasing human lifespan is complicated and has important ethical ramifications. While there may be advantages to living longer, it is crucial to take into account the larger social and philosophical ramifications before *creating life-extension technologies.*

***How long-lived women affect society and the economy**

The extended life expectancy of women has a substantial impact on the economy and society in different ways. More women are working longer because they are living longer than ever before. Because more people are working and contributing to productivity and economic growth, there is a positive effect on the economy from this increased labor participation. Women tend to live longer, which means that in addition to caring for their spouses and kids, women frequently look after their elderly parents as well. Caregiving obligations can harm women's ability to work and earn money, which can have a big impact on family dynamics and the economy. Women are more likely to need healthcare services as they get older and live longer than men do. As the population ages, healthcare expenses are therefore predicted to increase, and the longer lifespan of women is a factor in this development. The longer lifespan of women necessitates lengthier retirement planning for them. As well as the social security and pension systems, this has ramifications for retirement planning and savings. Since women often outlive males, they have more time to spend money on goods and services. Women are also more likely to be the principal consumers in many households.

Women's longevity has a tremendous impact on society and the economy, affecting everything from employment involvement and family dynamics to healthcare costs and retirement planning. This can be beneficial to the economy because it creates demand for goods and services. Planning for the future of society and the economy must take the implications of women's longevity into account.

Conclusion

The intricacy of the issue of women's longevity is influenced by a variety of factors, including biological, nutritional, behavioral, cultural, and social ones. By being mindful of these factors, we may be able to take action to improve the health and wellness of women and possibly lengthen their lives. In almost all current populations, women currently outlive males. While some studies emphasize the social influences' importance, others concentrate on the biological causes of the female advantage. In populations of slaves and populations that had experienced severe famines and epidemics, *inequalities between male-female survivorship.* We discovered that women survived longer on average than males even when mortality was relatively high. *The majority of the female advantage resulted from gender-specific differences in infant mortality; baby* girls fared better under difficult circumstances than baby males. These findings are consistent with the hypothesis that the female survival advantage is influenced by a complex interplay between biological, environmental, and social factors. Even though females often outlive males across all species, mortality risk does not rise as quickly in males as it does in females. Consequently, they assert, there must be additional, more complicated elements at work, such as the animals' living environments and sex-specific development, survival, and reproduction over the history of the species. For instance, traveling males may be exposed to more infections in the environment, according to certain research. Three populations of bighorn sheep were affected by this. *Local environmental factors that compromise reproduction and survival may also have an impact on the size of the lifespan disparity.* In some animals, males devote more energy to mating and reproduction, which could result in greater lifespan disparities between the sexes, according to scientists. Female survival rises when males supply some or all of the parental care, which is another explanation for the sex difference. If both parents contribute to raising their children, the expense of giving birth and caring for the young decreases, which is good for female health. The data on wild animals will be compared with the data on mammals maintained in zoos, where they are not required to engage in combat with predators, compete for food, or marry, to determine the extent to which biological variations between the sexes' affect life expectancy.s The results are anticipated to help researchers better understand the factors that influence human longevity. *Humans now live longer on average than they did a century ago thanks to better living conditions and medical advancements. The fact that women continue to outlive men suggests that biological differences also play a part in longevity.* The U.S. Centers for Disease Control predict that the typical American man will live to be an average of 75 years old and the average American woman will live to be over 80 years old. Women can anticipate living longer and being in better health than males. According to experts, biological and social variables are to blame for the gap. As men age, their immune systems weaken and their risk of cardiovascular diseases increases, which are both related to the hormone testosterone in men. It is also connected to dangerous behaviors including *drinking, smoking, and eating unhealthily.* Men are less likely than women to heed a doctor's instructions after a diagnosis. According to statistics, men are more prone to engage in life-threatening activities and perish in vehicle accidents or gunfights. According to a recent study from a hospital in Zurich, intricate interplay between regional environmental factors and sex-specific reproductive biology are what determine the disparities in longevity between men and women. It is predicted that further study will yield "innovative insights into the evolutionary roots and physiology underlying aging in both sexes."

Women are known to live longer than men, and this has been the subject of extensive study and conjecture. Others say it has to do with genetics or lifestyle issues, while some think it's because women often take better care of their health. Several little-known factors contribute to women's longevity, though. **The strength of community** is one of the keys to women's lifespan. It has been demonstrated that women tend to have better social ties than men, which benefits their health and well-being. According to studies, women with robust social networks live longer than those who are more socially isolated. This is because a caring community can aid in lowering stress, elevating mood, and encouraging healthy behaviors. **A nutritious diet is another key to women living longer.** Women are more likely to maintain a balanced and nutritious diet since they are generally more conscious of what they consume. This can aid in lowering the risk of chronic illnesses including cancer, diabetes, and heart disease, which can have a serious negative impact on life expectancy. **Another factor contributing to women's longevity is regular exercise**. The fact that women are often more active than males can have a big impact on their general health and well-being. Exercise can enhance mood and cognitive function, lower the chance of developing chronic diseases, and support healthy aging. **Another key to women's longevity is their emotional toughness**, which is well documented. Women often express their emotions more than males do, which can make it easier for them to handle stress and misfortune. Women who exhibit high levels of emotional resilience are more likely to live longer and enjoy greater general health, according to studies. **Finally, women who have an optimistic outlook tend to live longer**. Women are more likely to have a more upbeat attitude toward life and perceive things as half full rather than half empty. By doing so, they may be able to handle stress more effectively, lower their chance of developing depression, and generally feel better.